Your Food Diary

Three Month Edition

By Greg W. Steinacker

© 2011 Greg W. Steinacker

**This book is meant to be used in conjunction with a healthy diet and exercise plan to assist you in losing weight and monitoring your blood sugar levels. Remember to consult your doctor before starting any new diet or exercise plan.

ISBN-13: 978-1453639016

ISBN-10: 1453639012

BISAC: Health & Fitness / General

There are eight Sections on each page and there is a "notes" page for each week to record anything you think will help you:

Breakfast - Write what you have for breakfast here. Also contains a place to record the time you finish a meal as well as a Fasting Glucose Level (FAST GL) and a GL for 2 hours (GL@2HRS) after the meal.

Snack - Write what you have for snack here if you have one.

Lunch - Write what you have for lunch here. Also contains a place to record the time you finish a meal as well as a GL@2HRS.

Snack - Write what you have for snack here if you have one.

Dinner - Write what you have for dinner here. Also contains a place to record the time you finish a meal as well as a GL@2HRS.

Snack - Write what you have for snack here if you have one.

Water - For recording the number of 8 oz. glasses of water you have per day. (Water only, other beverages should go under the meal or snack you have them with.)

Exercise - Write what exercises you do here. There is a spot here to record your heart rate after exercise.

On Sundays, there is a place for you to record your weight making it easier to keep track of your weight loss/gain.

Diet and Exercise Tips:

- Weigh yourself in the morning as soon as you get up. You are lighter in the morning than at night.

- Do not weigh yourself daily, only weekly or bi-weekly. You weight will fluctuate and weighing yourself daily can get discouraging.

- Do not eat canned or processed foods. If you don't know what an ingredient is, you probably shouldn't be eating it. Soups and stews you make at home are better for you than anything that comes out of a can, and they taste better because you control the ingredients.

- Buy fresh or frozen fruits and veggies instead of canned, better yet, grow some of them yourself if you can. Fresh and frozen fruits and veggies are better for you.

- Keep a positive attitude. Everyone falters and no one is perfect. Don't give up!

- Take a sanity break and have a dessert once in a while. Just be realistic.

- Exercise is important, but don't overdo it. You don't want to lose ground because of an injury.

- Muscle burns energy. Try to strengthen your entire body as well as your cardiovascular system.

- Housework IS exercise, but with today's household appliances, it is not enough on its own.

- Take 10,000 steps a day. It is as easy as putting one foot in front of the other.

Date:

Breakfast (Time -)		Fasting GL	
		Time	
		GL@2HRS	
		Time	

Snack:

Lunch (Time -)			
		GL@2HRS	
		Time	

Snack:

Dinner (Time -)			
		GL@2HRS	
		Time	

Snack:

Water:	Exercise:	Heart Rate:	
		Weight:	

Date: _____

Breakfast (Time -)		Fasting GL	
		Time	
		GL@2HRS	
		Time	

Snack:

Lunch (Time -)			
		GL@2HRS	
		Time	

Snack:

Dinner (Time -)			
		GL@2HRS	
		Time	

Snack:

Water:	Exercise:	Heart Rate:	

Date:

Breakfast (Time -   )

Fasting GL	
Time	

GL@2HRS	
Time	

Snack:

Lunch (Time -   )

GL@2HRS	
Time	

Snack:

Dinner (Time -   )

GL@2HRS	
Time	

Snack:

Water:	**Exercise:**	Heart Rate:	

Date:

Breakfast (Time -   )

Fasting GL	
Time	

GL@2HRS	
Time	

Snack:

Lunch (Time -   )

GL@2HRS	
Time	

Snack:

Dinner (Time -   )

GL@2HRS	
Time	

Snack:

Water:	**Exercise:**	**Heart Rate:**	

Date:

Breakfast (Time -)		Fasting GL	
		Time	
		GL@2HRS	
		Time	

Snack:

Lunch (Time -)			
		GL@2HRS	
		Time	

Snack:

Dinner (Time -)			
		GL@2HRS	
		Time	

Snack:

Water:	Exercise:	Heart Rate:	

Date:

Breakfast (Time -)		Fasting GL	
		Time	
		GL@2HRS	
		Time	

Snack:

Lunch (Time -)			
		GL@2HRS	
		Time	

Snack:

Dinner (Time -)			
		GL@2HRS	
		Time	

Snack:

Water:	Exercise:	Heart Rate:	

Date:

Breakfast (Time -   )

	Fasting GL	
	Time	

	GL@2HRS	
	Time	

Snack:

Lunch (Time -   )

	GL@2HRS	
	Time	

Snack:

Dinner (Time -   )

	GL@2HRS	
	Time	

Snack:

Water:	**Exercise:**	Heart Rate:	

Date:

Breakfast (Time -)		Fasting GL	
		Time	
		GL@2HRS	
		Time	

Snack:

Lunch (Time -)			
		GL@2HRS	
		Time	

Snack:

Dinner (Time -)			
		GL@2HRS	
		Time	

Snack:

Water:	Exercise:	Heart Rate:	
		Weight:	

Date:

Breakfast (Time -   )   **Fasting GL**

                                                                        Time

                                                                        GL@2HRS

                                                                        Time

Snack:

Lunch (Time -   )

                                                                        GL@2HRS

                                                                        Time

Snack:

Dinner (Time -   )

                                                                        GL@2HRS

                                                                        Time

Snack:

Water: **Exercise:**   **Heart Rate:**

Date:

Breakfast (Time -)	Fasting GL	
	Time	
	GL@2HRS	
	Time	

Snack:

Lunch (Time -)		
	GL@2HRS	
	Time	

Snack:

Dinner (Time -)		
	GL@2HRS	
	Time	

Snack:

Water:	Exercise:	Heart Rate:	

Date:

Breakfast (Time -)		Fasting GL	
		Time	
		GL@2HRS	
		Time	

Snack:

Lunch (Time -)			
		GL@2HRS	
		Time	

Snack:

Dinner (Time -)			
		GL@2HRS	
		Time	

Snack:

Water:	Exercise:	Heart Rate:	

Date:

Breakfast (Time -   )

Fasting GL	
Time	

GL@2HRS	
Time	

Snack:

Lunch (Time -   )

GL@2HRS	
Time	

Snack:

Dinner (Time -   )

GL@2HRS	
Time	

Snack:

Water:	**Exercise:**	**Heart Rate:**	

Date:

Breakfast (Time -)		Fasting GL	
		Time	
		GL@2HRS	
		Time	

Snack:

Lunch (Time -)			
		GL@2HRS	
		Time	

Snack:

Dinner (Time -)			
		GL@2HRS	
		Time	

Snack:

Water:	Exercise:	Heart Rate:	

Date:

Breakfast (Time -)	Fasting GL	
	Time	
	GL@2HRS	
	Time	

Snack:

Lunch (Time -)		
	GL@2HRS	
	Time	

Snack:

Dinner (Time -)		
	GL@2HRS	
	Time	

Snack:

| Water: | Exercise: | Heart Rate: | |

Date:

Breakfast (Time -)		Fasting GL	
		Time	
		GL@2HRS	
		Time	

Snack:

Lunch (Time -)			
		GL@2HRS	
		Time	

Snack:

Dinner (Time -)			
		GL@2HRS	
		Time	

Snack:

Water:	Exercise:	Heart Rate:	
		Weight:	

Date:

Breakfast (Time -)		**Fasting GL**	
		Time	
		GL@2HRS	
		Time	

Snack:

Lunch (Time -)			
		GL@2HRS	
		Time	

Snack:

Dinner (Time -)			
		GL@2HRS	
		Time	

Snack:

| **Water:** | **Exercise:** | **Heart Rate:** | |

Date:

Breakfast (Time -   )

Fasting GL	
Time	

GL@2HRS	
Time	

Snack:

Lunch (Time -   )

GL@2HRS	
Time	

Snack:

Dinner (Time -   )

GL@2HRS	
Time	

Snack:

Water:	Exercise:	Heart Rate:	

Date:

Breakfast (Time -)		Fasting GL	
		Time	
		GL@2HRS	
		Time	

Snack:

Lunch (Time -)			
		GL@2HRS	
		Time	

Snack:

Dinner (Time -)			
		GL@2HRS	
		Time	

Snack:

Water:	Exercise:	Heart Rate:	

Date:

Breakfast (Time -)		Fasting GL	
		Time	
		GL@2HRS	
		Time	

Snack:

Lunch (Time -)			
		GL@2HRS	
		Time	

Snack:

Dinner (Time -)			
		GL@2HRS	
		Time	

Snack:

Water:	Exercise:	Heart Rate:	

Date:

Breakfast (Time -   )

	Fasting GL	
	Time	

	GL@2HRS	
	Time	

Snack:

Lunch (Time -   )

	GL@2HRS	
	Time	

Snack:

Dinner (Time -   )

	GL@2HRS	
	Time	

Snack:

Water:	**Exercise:**	**Heart Rate:**	

Date:

Breakfast (Time -   )

Fasting GL	
Time	

GL@2HRS	
Time	

Snack:

Lunch (Time -   )

GL@2HRS	
Time	

Snack:

Dinner (Time -   )

GL@2HRS	
Time	

Snack:

Water:	**Exercise:**	Heart Rate:	

Date:

Breakfast (Time -)		Fasting GL	
		Time	
		GL@2HRS	
		Time	

Snack:

Lunch (Time -)		GL@2HRS	
		Time	

Snack:

Dinner (Time -)		GL@2HRS	
		Time	

Snack:

Water:	Exercise:	Heart Rate:	
		Weight:	

Date:

Breakfast (Time -   )

Fasting GL	
Time	

GL@2HRS	
Time	

Snack:

Lunch (Time -   )

GL@2HRS	
Time	

Snack:

Dinner (Time -   )

GL@2HRS	
Time	

Snack:

Water:	**Exercise:**	**Heart Rate:**	

Date:

Breakfast (Time -)	Fasting GL	
	Time	
	GL@2HRS	
	Time	

Snack:

Lunch (Time -)		
	GL@2HRS	
	Time	

Snack:

Dinner (Time -)		
	GL@2HRS	
	Time	

Snack:

Water:	**Exercise:**	Heart Rate:	

Date:

Breakfast (Time -)		Fasting GL	
		Time	
		GL@2HRS	
		Time	

Snack:

Lunch (Time -)			
		GL@2HRS	
		Time	

Snack:

Dinner (Time -)			
		GL@2HRS	
		Time	

Snack:

Water:	Exercise:	Heart Rate:	

Date:

Breakfast (Time -)		Fasting GL	
		Time	
		GL@2HRS	
		Time	

Snack:

Lunch (Time -)			
		GL@2HRS	
		Time	

Snack:

Dinner (Time -)			
		GL@2HRS	
		Time	

Snack:

Water:	Exercise:	Heart Rate:	

Date:

Breakfast (Time -)		Fasting GL	
		Time	
		GL@2HRS	
		Time	

Snack:

Lunch (Time -)			
		GL@2HRS	
		Time	

Snack:

Dinner (Time -)			
		GL@2HRS	
		Time	

Snack:

Water:	Exercise:	Heart Rate:	

Date:

Breakfast (Time -)		Fasting GL	
		Time	
		GL@2HRS	
		Time	

Snack:

Lunch (Time -)			
		GL@2HRS	
		Time	

Snack:

Dinner (Time -)			
		GL@2HRS	
		Time	

Snack:

Water:	Exercise:	Heart Rate:	

Date:

Breakfast (Time -   )

Fasting GL	
Time	

GL@2HRS	
Time	

Snack:

Lunch (Time -   )

GL@2HRS	
Time	

Snack:

Dinner (Time -   )

GL@2HRS	
Time	

Snack:

Water:	**Exercise:**	Heart Rate:	
		Weight:	

Date:

Breakfast (Time -)		Fasting GL	
		Time	
		GL@2HRS	
		Time	

Snack:

Lunch (Time -)			
		GL@2HRS	
		Time	

Snack:

Dinner (Time -)			
		GL@2HRS	
		Time	

Snack:

Water:	Exercise:	Heart Rate:	

Date:

Breakfast (Time -)		Fasting GL	
		Time	
		GL@2HRS	
		Time	

Snack:

Lunch (Time -)			
		GL@2HRS	
		Time	

Snack:

Dinner (Time -)			
		GL@2HRS	
		Time	

Snack:

Water:	Exercise:	Heart Rate:	

Date:

Breakfast (Time -)		Fasting GL	
		Time	
		GL@2HRS	
		Time	

| Snack: | | | |

Lunch (Time -)			
		GL@2HRS	
		Time	

| Snack: | | | |

Dinner (Time -)			
		GL@2HRS	
		Time	

| Snack: | | | |

| Water: | Exercise: | Heart Rate: | |

Date:

Breakfast (Time -   )

Fasting GL	
Time	
GL@2HRS	
Time	

Snack:

Lunch (Time -   )

GL@2HRS	
Time	

Snack:

Dinner (Time -   )

GL@2HRS	
Time	

Snack:

Water:	**Exercise:**	Heart Rate:	

Date:

Breakfast (Time -)		Fasting GL	
		Time	
		GL@2HRS	
		Time	

Snack:

Lunch (Time -)			
		GL@2HRS	
		Time	

Snack:

Dinner (Time -)			
		GL@2HRS	
		Time	

Snack:

Water:	Exercise:	Heart Rate:	

Date:

Breakfast (Time -)	Fasting GL	
	Time	
	GL@2HRS	
	Time	

| Snack: |
| |

Lunch (Time -)		
	GL@2HRS	
	Time	

| Snack: |
| |

Dinner (Time -)		
	GL@2HRS	
	Time	

| Snack: |
| |

| Water: | Exercise: | Heart Rate: |

Date:

Breakfast (Time -)	Fasting GL	
	Time	
	GL@2HRS	
	Time	

Snack:

Lunch (Time -)		
	GL@2HRS	
	Time	

Snack:

Dinner (Time -)		
	GL@2HRS	
	Time	

Snack:

Water:	Exercise:	Heart Rate:	
		Weight:	

Date:

Breakfast (Time -)		Fasting GL	
		Time	
		GL@2HRS	
		Time	

Snack:

Lunch (Time -)			
		GL@2HRS	
		Time	

Snack:

Dinner (Time -)			
		GL@2HRS	
		Time	

Snack:

Water:	Exercise:	Heart Rate:	

Date:

Breakfast (Time -)	Fasting GL	
	Time	
	GL@2HRS	
	Time	

Snack:

Lunch (Time -)		
	GL@2HRS	
	Time	

Snack:

Dinner (Time -)		
	GL@2HRS	
	Time	

Snack:

| Water: | Exercise: | Heart Rate: | |

Date:

Breakfast (Time -   )

Fasting GL	
Time	

GL@2HRS	
Time	

Snack:

Lunch (Time -   )

GL@2HRS	
Time	

Snack:

Dinner (Time -   )

GL@2HRS	
Time	

Snack:

Water:	**Exercise:**	**Heart Rate:**	

Date:

Breakfast (Time -)		Fasting GL	
		Time	
		GL@2HRS	
		Time	

Snack:

Lunch (Time -)			
		GL@2HRS	
		Time	

Snack:

Dinner (Time -)			
		GL@2HRS	
		Time	

Snack:

Water:	Exercise:	Heart Rate:	

Date: _____

Breakfast (Time -   )

| | Fasting GL | |
| | Time | |

| | GL@2HRS | |
| | Time | |

Snack:

Lunch (Time -   )

| | GL@2HRS | |
| | Time | |

Snack:

Dinner (Time -   )

| | GL@2HRS | |
| | Time | |

Snack:

| **Water:** | **Exercise:** | Heart Rate: | |

Date:

Breakfast (Time -)		Fasting GL	
		Time	
		GL@2HRS	
		Time	

Snack:

Lunch (Time -)			
		GL@2HRS	
		Time	

Snack:

Dinner (Time -)			
		GL@2HRS	
		Time	

Snack:

Water:	Exercise:	Heart Rate:	

Date:

Breakfast (Time -   )

Fasting GL	
Time	

GL@2HRS	
Time	

Snack:

Lunch (Time -   )

GL@2HRS	
Time	

Snack:

Dinner (Time -   )

GL@2HRS	
Time	

Snack:

Water:	**Exercise:**	Heart Rate:	
		Weight:	

Date:

Breakfast (Time -)		Fasting GL	
		Time	
		GL@2HRS	
		Time	

Snack:

Lunch (Time -)			
		GL@2HRS	
		Time	

Snack:

Dinner (Time -)			
		GL@2HRS	
		Time	

Snack:

Water:	Exercise:	Heart Rate:	

Date:

Breakfast (Time -)	Fasting GL	
	Time	
	GL@2HRS	
	Time	

| Snack: |
| |

Lunch (Time -)		
	GL@2HRS	
	Time	

| Snack: |
| |

Dinner (Time -)		
	GL@2HRS	
	Time	

| Snack: |
| |

| Water: | Exercise: | Heart Rate: | |
| | | |

Date:

Breakfast (Time -)	Fasting GL	
	Time	
	GL@2HRS	
	Time	

Snack:

Lunch (Time -)		
	GL@2HRS	
	Time	

Snack:

Dinner (Time -)		
	GL@2HRS	
	Time	

Snack:

| Water: | Exercise: | Heart Rate: | |

Date:

Breakfast (Time -)	Fasting GL	
	Time	
	GL@2HRS	
	Time	

Snack:

Lunch (Time -)	
	GL@2HRS	
	Time	

Snack:

Dinner (Time -)	
	GL@2HRS	
	Time	

Snack:

Water:	**Exercise:**	Heart Rate:	

Date:

Breakfast (Time -)	Fasting GL	
	Time	
	GL@2HRS	
	Time	

| Snack: |

| Lunch (Time -   ) |
| | GL@2HRS | |
| | Time | |

| Snack: |

| Dinner (Time -   ) |
| | GL@2HRS | |
| | Time | |

| Snack: |

| Water: | Exercise: | Heart Rate: | |

Date:

Breakfast (Time -)		Fasting GL	
		Time	
		GL@2HRS	
		Time	

Snack:

Lunch (Time -)			
		GL@2HRS	
		Time	

Snack:

Dinner (Time -)			
		GL@2HRS	
		Time	

Snack:

Water:	Exercise:	Heart Rate:	

Eat Healthy, Exercise Often

Date:

Breakfast (Time -   )

Fasting GL	
Time	

GL@2HRS	
Time	

Snack:

Lunch (Time -   )

GL@2HRS	
Time	

Snack:

Dinner (Time -   )

GL@2HRS	
Time	

Snack:

Water:	**Exercise:**	Heart Rate:	
		Weight:	

Date:

Breakfast (Time -   )

	Fasting GL	
	Time	

	GL@2HRS	
	Time	

Snack:

Lunch (Time -   )

	GL@2HRS	
	Time	

Snack:

Dinner (Time -   )

	GL@2HRS	
	Time	

Snack:

Water:	**Exercise:**	**Heart Rate:**	

Date:

Breakfast (Time -)	Fasting GL	
	Time	
	GL@2HRS	
	Time	

| Snack: |
| |

Lunch (Time -)		
	GL@2HRS	
	Time	

| Snack: |
| |

Dinner (Time -)		
	GL@2HRS	
	Time	

| Snack: |
| |

| Water: | Exercise: | Heart Rate: | |

Date:

Breakfast (Time -)	Fasting GL	
	Time	
	GL@2HRS	
	Time	

| Snack: |

Lunch (Time -)	
	GL@2HRS	
	Time	

| Snack: |

Dinner (Time -)	
	GL@2HRS	
	Time	

| Snack: |

| Water: | Exercise: | Heart Rate: |

Date:

Breakfast (Time -   )

| Fasting GL | |
| Time | |

| GL@2HRS | |
| Time | |

Snack:

Lunch (Time -   )

| GL@2HRS | |
| Time | |

Snack:

Dinner (Time -   )

| GL@2HRS | |
| Time | |

Snack:

| Water: | Exercise: | Heart Rate: | |

Date:

Breakfast (Time -)		Fasting GL	
		Time	
		GL@2HRS	
		Time	

Snack:

Lunch (Time -)			
		GL@2HRS	
		Time	

Snack:

Dinner (Time -)			
		GL@2HRS	
		Time	

Snack:

Water:	Exercise:	Heart Rate:	

Date:

Breakfast (Time -   )

Fasting GL	
Time	

GL@2HRS	
Time	

Snack:

Lunch (Time -   )

GL@2HRS	
Time	

Snack:

Dinner (Time -   )

GL@2HRS	
Time	

Snack:

Water:	Exercise:	Heart Rate:	

Date:

Breakfast (Time -)		Fasting GL	
		Time	
		GL@2HRS	
		Time	
Snack:			
Lunch (Time -)			
		GL@2HRS	
		Time	
Snack:			
Dinner (Time -)			
		GL@2HRS	
		Time	
Snack:			

| Water: | Exercise: | Heart Rate: | |
| | | Weight: | |

Date:

Breakfast (Time -)		Fasting GL	
		Time	
		GL@2HRS	
		Time	

Snack:

Lunch (Time -)			
		GL@2HRS	
		Time	

Snack:

Dinner (Time -)			
		GL@2HRS	
		Time	

Snack:

Water:	Exercise:	Heart Rate:	

Date:

Breakfast (Time -)		Fasting GL	
		Time	
		GL@2HRS	
		Time	

Snack:

Lunch (Time -)			
		GL@2HRS	
		Time	

Snack:

Dinner (Time -)			
		GL@2HRS	
		Time	

Snack:

Water:	Exercise:	Heart Rate:	

Date:

Breakfast (Time -   ) | Fasting GL |
| Time |

| GL@2HRS |
| Time |

Snack:

Lunch (Time -   )

| GL@2HRS |
| Time |

Snack:

Dinner (Time -   )

| GL@2HRS |
| Time |

Snack:

Water: | **Exercise:** | **Heart Rate:** |

Date:

Breakfast (Time -)		Fasting GL	
		Time	
		GL@2HRS	
		Time	

Snack:

Lunch (Time -)			
		GL@2HRS	
		Time	

Snack:

Dinner (Time -)			
		GL@2HRS	
		Time	

Snack:

| Water: | Exercise: | Heart Rate: | |

Date:

Breakfast (Time -)		Fasting GL	
		Time	
		GL@2HRS	
		Time	

Snack:

Lunch (Time -)			
		GL@2HRS	
		Time	

Snack:

Dinner (Time -)			
		GL@2HRS	
		Time	

Snack:

Water:	Exercise:	Heart Rate:	

Date:

Breakfast (Time -)		Fasting GL	
		Time	
		GL@2HRS	
		Time	

Snack:			

Lunch (Time -)			
		GL@2HRS	
		Time	

Snack:			

Dinner (Time -)			
		GL@2HRS	
		Time	

Snack:			

Water:	Exercise:	Heart Rate:	

Date:

Breakfast (Time -)		Fasting GL	
		Time	
		GL@2HRS	
		Time	

Snack:

Lunch (Time -)			
		GL@2HRS	
		Time	

Snack:

Dinner (Time -)			
		GL@2HRS	
		Time	

Snack:

Water:	Exercise:	Heart Rate:	
		Weight:	

Date:

Breakfast (Time -   )

Fasting GL	
Time	
GL@2HRS	
Time	

Snack:

Lunch (Time -   )

GL@2HRS	
Time	

Snack:

Dinner (Time -   )

GL@2HRS	
Time	

Snack:

Water:	**Exercise:**	Heart Rate:	

Date:

Breakfast (Time -)		Fasting GL	
		Time	
		GL@2HRS	
		Time	

Snack:

Lunch (Time -)			
		GL@2HRS	
		Time	

Snack:

Dinner (Time -)			
		GL@2HRS	
		Time	

Snack:

Water:	Exercise:	Heart Rate:	

Date:

Breakfast (Time -   )

	Fasting GL	
	Time	

	GL@2HRS	
	Time	

Snack:

Lunch (Time -   )

	GL@2HRS	
	Time	

Snack:

Dinner (Time -   )

	GL@2HRS	
	Time	

Snack:

Water:	**Exercise:**	Heart Rate:	

Date:

Breakfast (Time -   )

Fasting GL	
Time	
GL@2HRS	
Time	

Snack:

Lunch (Time -   )

GL@2HRS	
Time	

Snack:

Dinner (Time -   )

GL@2HRS	
Time	

Snack:

Water:	**Exercise:**	Heart Rate:

Date:

Breakfast (Time -)		Fasting GL	
		Time	
		GL@2HRS	
		Time	

Snack:

Lunch (Time -)			
		GL@2HRS	
		Time	

Snack:

Dinner (Time -)			
		GL@2HRS	
		Time	

Snack:

Water:	Exercise:	Heart Rate:	

Date:

Breakfast (Time -)		Fasting GL	
		Time	
		GL@2HRS	
		Time	

Snack:

Lunch (Time -)			
		GL@2HRS	
		Time	

Snack:

Dinner (Time -)			
		GL@2HRS	
		Time	

Snack:

Water:	Exercise:	Heart Rate:	

Date:

Breakfast (Time -)		Fasting GL	
		Time	
		GL@2HRS	
		Time	

Snack:

Lunch (Time -)			
		GL@2HRS	
		Time	

Snack:

Dinner (Time -)			
		GL@2HRS	
		Time	

Snack:

Water:	Exercise:	Heart Rate:	
		Weight:	

Date:

Breakfast (Time -   )

Fasting GL

Time

GL@2HRS

Time

Snack:

Lunch (Time -   )

GL@2HRS

Time

Snack:

Dinner (Time -   )

GL@2HRS

Time

Snack:

Water:

Exercise:

Heart Rate:

Date:

Breakfast (Time -)		Fasting GL	
		Time	
		GL@2HRS	
		Time	

Snack:

Lunch (Time -)			
		GL@2HRS	
		Time	

Snack:

Dinner (Time -)			
		GL@2HRS	
		Time	

Snack:

Water:	Exercise:	Heart Rate:	

Date:

Breakfast (Time -)	Fasting GL	
	Time	
	GL@2HRS	
	Time	

Snack:

Lunch (Time -)	GL@2HRS	
	Time	

Snack:

Dinner (Time -)	GL@2HRS	
	Time	

Snack:

Water:	Exercise:	Heart Rate:	

Date:

Breakfast (Time -)		Fasting GL	
		Time	
		GL@2HRS	
		Time	

Snack:

Lunch (Time -)			
		GL@2HRS	
		Time	

Snack:

Dinner (Time -)			
		GL@2HRS	
		Time	

Snack:

Water:	Exercise:	Heart Rate:	

Date:

Breakfast (Time -)		Fasting GL	
		Time	
		GL@2HRS	
		Time	

Snack:

Lunch (Time -)			
		GL@2HRS	
		Time	

Snack:

Dinner (Time -)			
		GL@2HRS	
		Time	

Snack:

| Water: | Exercise: | Heart Rate: | |

Date:

Breakfast (Time -)		Fasting GL	
		Time	
		GL@2HRS	
		Time	

Snack:

Lunch (Time -)			
		GL@2HRS	
		Time	

Snack:

Dinner (Time -)			
		GL@2HRS	
		Time	

Snack:

Water:	Exercise:	Heart Rate:	

Date:

Breakfast (Time -   )

Fasting GL	
Time	
GL@2HRS	
Time	

Snack:

Lunch (Time -   )

GL@2HRS	
Time	

Snack:

Dinner (Time -   )

GL@2HRS	
Time	

Snack:

Water:	**Exercise:**	Heart Rate:	
		Weight:	

Date:

Breakfast (Time -)		Fasting GL	
		Time	
		GL@2HRS	
		Time	

Snack:

Lunch (Time -)			
		GL@2HRS	
		Time	

Snack:

Dinner (Time -)			
		GL@2HRS	
		Time	

Snack:

Water:	Exercise:	Heart Rate:	

Date:

Breakfast (Time -)	Fasting GL	
	Time	
	GL@2HRS	
	Time	

Snack:

Lunch (Time -)		
	GL@2HRS	
	Time	

Snack:

Dinner (Time -)		
	GL@2HRS	
	Time	

Snack:

Water:	Exercise:	Heart Rate:	

Date:

Breakfast (Time -   )

| | Fasting GL | |
| | Time | |

| | GL@2HRS | |
| | Time | |

Snack:

Lunch (Time -   )

| | GL@2HRS | |
| | Time | |

Snack:

Dinner (Time -   )

| | GL@2HRS | |
| | Time | |

Snack:

| **Water:** | **Exercise:** | **Heart Rate:** | |

Date:

Breakfast (Time -)	Fasting GL	
	Time	
	GL@2HRS	
	Time	

Snack:

Lunch (Time -)		
	GL@2HRS	
	Time	

Snack:

Dinner (Time -)		
	GL@2HRS	
	Time	

Snack:

Water:	Exercise:	Heart Rate:

Date:

Breakfast (Time -)		Fasting GL	
		Time	
		GL@2HRS	
		Time	

Snack:

Lunch (Time -)			
		GL@2HRS	
		Time	

Snack:

Dinner (Time -)			
		GL@2HRS	
		Time	

Snack:

Water:	Exercise:	Heart Rate:	

Date:

Breakfast (Time -)	Fasting GL	
	Time	
	GL@2HRS	
	Time	

Snack:

Lunch (Time -)		
	GL@2HRS	
	Time	

Snack:

Dinner (Time -)		
	GL@2HRS	
	Time	

Snack:

Water:	Exercise:	Heart Rate:	

Date:

Breakfast (Time -)	Fasting GL	
	Time	
	GL@2HRS	
	Time	

Snack:

Lunch (Time -)		
	GL@2HRS	
	Time	

Snack:

Dinner (Time -)		
	GL@2HRS	
	Time	

Snack:

Water:	Exercise:	Heart Rate:
		Weight:

Date:

Breakfast (Time -)	Fasting GL	
	Time	
	GL@2HRS	
	Time	

Snack:

Lunch (Time -)		
	GL@2HRS	
	Time	

Snack:

Dinner (Time -)		
	GL@2HRS	
	Time	

Snack:

Water:	Exercise:	Heart Rate:	

Date:

Breakfast (Time -)		Fasting GL	
		Time	
		GL@2HRS	
		Time	

Snack:

Lunch (Time -)			
		GL@2HRS	
		Time	

Snack:

Dinner (Time -)			
		GL@2HRS	
		Time	

Snack:

Water:	Exercise:	Heart Rate:	

Date:

Breakfast (Time -)	Fasting GL	
	Time	
	GL@2HRS	
	Time	

Snack:

Lunch (Time -)		
	GL@2HRS	
	Time	

Snack:

Dinner (Time -)		
	GL@2HRS	
	Time	

Snack:

| Water: | Exercise: | Heart Rate: |

Date:

Breakfast (Time -)		Fasting GL	
		Time	
		GL@2HRS	
		Time	

Snack:			

Lunch (Time -)			
		GL@2HRS	
		Time	

Snack:			

Dinner (Time -)			
		GL@2HRS	
		Time	

Snack:			

Water:	Exercise:	Heart Rate:	

Date:

Breakfast (Time -)	Fasting GL	
	Time	
	GL@2HRS	
	Time	

| Snack: |
| |

Lunch (Time -)		
	GL@2HRS	
	Time	

| Snack: |
| |

Dinner (Time -)		
	GL@2HRS	
	Time	

| Snack: |
| |

| Water: | Exercise: | Heart Rate: | |

Date:

Breakfast (Time -)		Fasting GL	
		Time	
		GL@2HRS	
		Time	

Snack:

Lunch (Time -)			
		GL@2HRS	
		Time	

Snack:

Dinner (Time -)			
		GL@2HRS	
		Time	

Snack:

Water:	Exercise:	Heart Rate:	

Date:

Breakfast (Time -)		Fasting GL	
		Time	
		GL@2HRS	
		Time	

Snack:

Lunch (Time -)			
		GL@2HRS	
		Time	

Snack:

Dinner (Time -)			
		GL@2HRS	
		Time	

Snack:

| Water: | Exercise: | Heart Rate: | |
| | | Weight: | |

Date:

Breakfast (Time -)		Fasting GL	
		Time	
		GL@2HRS	
		Time	

Snack:

Lunch (Time -)			
		GL@2HRS	
		Time	

Snack:

Dinner (Time -)			
		GL@2HRS	
		Time	

Snack:

Water:	Exercise:	Heart Rate:	

Date:

Breakfast (Time -)		Fasting GL	
		Time	
		GL@2HRS	
		Time	

Snack:

Lunch (Time -)			
		GL@2HRS	
		Time	

Snack:

Dinner (Time -)			
		GL@2HRS	
		Time	

Snack:

Water:	Exercise:	Heart Rate:	

Date:

Breakfast (Time -)		Fasting GL	
		Time	
		GL@2HRS	
		Time	

Snack:

Lunch (Time -)			
		GL@2HRS	
		Time	

Snack:

Dinner (Time -)			
		GL@2HRS	
		Time	

Snack:

Water:	Exercise:	Heart Rate:	

Date:

Breakfast (Time -)	Fasting GL	
	Time	
	GL@2HRS	
	Time	

| Snack: |
| |

Lunch (Time -)		
	GL@2HRS	
	Time	

| Snack: |
| |

Dinner (Time -)		
	GL@2HRS	
	Time	

| Snack: |
| |

| Water: | Exercise: | Heart Rate: |
| | | |

Date:

Breakfast (Time -)	Fasting GL	
	Time	
	GL@2HRS	
	Time	

Snack:

Lunch (Time -)		
	GL@2HRS	
	Time	

Snack:

Dinner (Time -)		
	GL@2HRS	
	Time	

Snack:

Water:	Exercise:	Heart Rate:

Date:

Breakfast (Time -)		Fasting GL	
		Time	
		GL@2HRS	
		Time	

Snack:

Lunch (Time -)			
		GL@2HRS	
		Time	

Snack:

Dinner (Time -)			
		GL@2HRS	
		Time	

Snack:

| Water: | Exercise: | Heart Rate: | |